Unloc

Fast and Easy Chair Yoga

for Seniors Over 60

Unlocking Vitality, Weight Reduction
and
Aging Gracefully

By

JANE POWERS

be copied, scanned, faxed, or retained in part or full without approval from the publisher or creator.

Table of Content

Introduction

The beautiful world of chair yoga is a hidden gem waiting to be discovered in a world that never seems to slow down. This yoga, however, is designed just for our seasoned seniors and is your passport to a livelier, more balanced, and all-around terrific life.

Picture this place where staying calm and working out are intertwined.

Finding inner serenity is a special ability and simple stretches offer you an amazing energy boost. Chair yoga is a fun technique that increases flexibility, calmness, and vitality. With each session, you get more engrossed, and your chair becomes a doorway to serenity and a surge of fresh vitality. It acts as your road map to long-term wellness and satisfaction. It serves as your guide to enduring good health and contentment.

Are you ready to start your adventure of self-discovery, energy, and the unbridled joy of chair yoga? **"FAST AND EASY CHAIR YOGA FOR SENIORS OVER 6O:**

Unlocking Vitality, Weight Ruduction and Aging Gracefully" is just one stretch away from being your next adventure. So prepare for a journey by fastening your seatbelt.

Chapter 1

Introducing Chair Yoga

Good day! Let's explore the amazing world of chair yoga, an excellent choice for seniors wishing to maintain their health and level of activity. We'll introduce you to chair yoga in this chapter, go over all of its advantages, and help you set up your space and gear.

Why Seniors Should Practice Chair Yoga

For several convincing reasons, chair yoga is a real game-changer for elders. It is quite mild on aging joints first and foremost. The thought of lying down on a regular yoga mat might be scary as our bodies age and lose some of their former flexibility. This issue is excellently addressed by chair yoga, which provides constant support and stability, similar to having a reliable and comfy workout partner right by your side.

The advantages of chair yoga go beyond health:

They also cover psychological and emotional health. This exercise has a significant impact on posture and balance, which significantly boosts one's confidence. Furthermore, due to its low-impact nature, it is open to people of all physical abilities and fitness levels. Chair yoga is inherently inclusive and everyone is welcome to take part in the joy of movement and relaxation.

Chair yoga's advantages

Let's now explore the many benefits that chair yoga has to offer. This exercise is well known for its capacity to increase circulation, muscle strength, and flexibility. Seniors should choose it since it offers a holistic workout that is easy on the body. Many people discover that chair yoga eases tension, lowers stress, and encourages relaxation, ultimately improving their physical and mental health.

Don't forget about the sense of camaraderie that chair yoga promotes either. It offers a special chance for people to interact socially, build relationships, and enjoy the benefits of staying active together. Therefore, chair yoga satisfies all of these needs and more, whether your objective is to improve your physical health, lower your stress level, or widen your social circle.

Setting Up Your Area and Equipment.

It's simple to get started with chair yoga. The only thing you require is a strong chair, preferably one without wheels, set on a flat, non-slip surface. You might want to keep a few props on hand, such as a cushion or a yoga block, for extra comfort and support. The secret to a successful chair yoga practice is, in fact, comfort.

You are ready to start your chair yoga journey now that the basics have been addressed. The versatility of chair yoga is what makes it so appealing to seniors of all fitness levels. So sit down and let's begin this educational and health-improving journey.

Chapter 2

Getting Started

You have arrived at the heart of your chair yoga journey. We're going to lay the foundation for your practice in this chapter by delving into vital warm-up exercises, mastering the skill of keeping proper posture in your chair, and developing vital breathing techniques.

Warm-Up Activities

It is essential to warm up those muscles before moving into the more challenging stretches and poses. Start by doing some light neck rolls while turning your head up and down and side to side. Rotate your shoulders, relax your wrists, and spend a short time softly rocking your hips. Your body responds to these movements as a pleasant wake-up call, telling you that it's time to move.

The Right Position in a Chair.

It's crucial to keep the right posture when doing chair yoga. Start by firmly placing both feet hip-width apart on the ground. Make sure your spine is neutral and that your back is straight. Your shoulders should be relaxed and should be placed comfortably apart from your ears. To use your core muscles, lean toward the edge of the chair, and make an effort to distribute your weight across both hips.

Breathing Methods

The core of yoga, and chair yoga is no exception, is effective breathing. Here are two basic breathing exercises that you can easily integrate into your routine:

Taking Deep Breaths: With your feet flat on the floor and your back straight, take a comfortable seat. On your chest and abdomen place one hand each. Deeply inhale through your nose, enabling your diaphragm to widen and your belly to rise. Exhale gradually out of your mouth.

This method aids in relaxation and stress reduction.

4-7-8 Technique.

You know, you take a silent inhalation for about **4** counts, then you hold it without making any noise for the remaining **7** counts. Following that, you exhale everything through your lips for **8** counts. It resembles a formula for doing chair yoga while unwinding, concentrating, and achieving nirvana. It will become second nature to you, much like those warm-up exercises we discussed earlier.

Those warm-up offers also serve as the equivalent of the pregame show for your chair yoga party. You wriggle your wrists, rock your hips, move your neck, and do a little shoulder dance. Your body is essentially signaling, "Hey, I'm ready for some yoga action!"

You'll be able to benefit from all that chair yoga has to offer once you get comfortable with these warm-up techniques, perfect your chair posture, and master the art of masterful breathing. Your chair is like your loyal ally on this voyage.

Chapter 3

Chair Yoga Exercise

We're about to get into the most enjoyable part of chair yoga: the exercises! We'll examine the first sub-category.

Upper Body Stretches.

You will feel more calm and relieved after performing these exercises.

A neck Roll.

This exercise will give your neck a mini-massage. Move your head forward and backward while gently angling it from side to side. These controlled, moderate motions help to loosen up the neck and increase flexibility. The beginning of your upper body stretches should start in this manner.

Shrugging shoulders.

Take a moment to lift your shoulders towards your ears before letting them go. For your shoulder muscles to relax, repeat this several times. A great method to relax and make room in your upper body is to shrug your shoulders.

The chest opener

Place your hands on the armrests of your chair while sitting comfortably on the floor with your feet flat. Deeply inhale, then softly move your chest forward to slightly arch your upper back. This extends the front of your shoulders and opens up your chest. Exhale as you settle back and take a neutral stance. This chest opener exercise encourages proper posture while releasing tension in your shoulders and chest.

Stretches for lower body, category 2

Okay, let's concentrate on some lower body stretches that will leave you feeling great. We're referring to thigh stretches, knee lifts, and ankle circles.

Ankle circles

Assist when your ankles are feeling particularly stiff.

Simply sit or stand how you like, and begin rotating your ankles in a circular motion as if you were sketching with your big toe.

It's sort of great because it stretches out those joints and makes your feet feel like they're having a little dance party.

knee raises

Let's speak about knee lifts now. It involves raising your knees to your chest. It doesn't matter whether you sit down or stand up straight for this one. As if marching in place, raise one knee as high as you can before switching to the other. fantastic for your balance and thighs.

Thigh stretch

Is all about, stretching out those thighs. As you get to your feet, you grip your backside ankle and pull it toward your butt. It resembles a flamingo stand in some ways but serves a purpose. This one is for your quadriceps and is quite useful after exercise.

So, yes, these stretches can help you feel more flexible and maintain excellent health in your lower body. When you feel like it, give them a try; your legs will appreciate it.

Chapter 4

Balance and Coordination

Balance and coordination are very important in the field of fitness. Everyone should be concerned about it for their health, you know? It's not only for the fancy gymnastics or dancing professionals.

Seated Leg Lifts

Although they may seem simple, seated leg lifts are rather cool. Simply sit down, extend your legs, and stand on one leg. Actively maintaining your balance is the key. So, it's not as simple as it seems.

Foot Taps

Foot taps are really straightforward but deceptively powerful. Standing erect, you just tap one foot in front of the other while alternating sides. It all comes down to testing your body's sense of location, and as we all know, your brain needs to communicate with your legs to prevent you from losing your balance. It resembles a little balancing dance in several ways.

Workouts to Strengthen the Core

Now, core workouts are totally important. Making your abdominal and lower back muscles strong is the goal of exercises like planks, Russian twists, and leg lifts. It's important to maintain stability and proper balance rather than merely having a beach-ready six-pack. Your core is quite crucial since it acts as the movement's command center.

In other words, don't neglect learning about balance and coordination. They're practical talents. You'll move better and feel more certain if you incorporate core exercises, sitting leg lifts, and foot tapping into your program. Whether you're a fitness expert or just someone who wants to maintain their fitness, these things are worth attempting.

Chapter 5

Relaxation and Meditation

Using guided relaxation methods is like getting help from someone to relax. A soothing voice instructs you on how to relax your body and let go of tension as you settle into a comfortable posture, close your eyes, and listen. It is like an instant mental vacation.

Being mindfully present in the moment is the key to meditation. You take a seat, close your eyes, and concentrate on your breathing, thoughts, and physical sensations. It involves inhabiting the present moment and refraining from making judgments. It is pretty tranquil, although it initially looks to be a cerebral exercise.

Breathwork for Stress Reduction

It seems easy to breathe, doesn't it? There is a method for achieving it, nevertheless, that is comparable to a stress-relieving magic performance. You take a steady, deep breath in, focusing on the inhale and exhale. It's a simple yet powerful method for de-stressing and relaxing. As though by clicking a button, your body and mind are reset.

The benefits to your mental and physical health of these mindfulness and relaxation techniques are undeniable. Whether you employ guided relaxation, mindfulness meditation, or just a few quiet, deep breaths, you are taking a break from the daily grind. The next time you need to relax, try one of them. You'll be grateful to your body and mind.

Chapter 6

Chair Yoga Drills

Therefore, chair yoga is still incredibly great even if you're not quite ready to go all out with a yoga mat and poses that resemble pretzels. Let's go further into these chair yoga poses:

10-Minute Daily routine

To relax your body and clear your mind in only 10 minutes, try a quick chair yoga routine. Sit down in a sturdy chair with your feet flat on the floor and take a long, deep breath. It serves as a discreet pause button during a hectic day. You'll start with some simple spine twists and side stretches to loosen up. After that, rest for a short while by doing some sitting meditation. Also, remember to roll your ankles to increase circulation. It's amazing how one little session can help you feel more comfortable.

20-Minute Energizing routine

A chair yoga routine is perfect if you have 20 minutes to spare. Things start calmly before getting a little livelier. Elevate your legs, tense your abs, and do sitting forward bends and shoulder rolls to relax. It gives your body a small mini-recharge. You'll be more energized and equipped to do everything on your to-do list.

30-Minute Full Body Workout

On days when you have some more time, try the 30-minute full-body chair yoga workout. This one covers every aspect. It is a thorough workout that targets all of your body's muscles, head to toe. You'll develop more strength, flexibility, and balance. You'll also spend some time in sitting postures, which will help you locate your center and act as a kind of mini-meditation.

These chair yoga routines seem like your personal yoga menu. You may decide which choice best satisfies your requirements and schedule. Therefore, whether you need a quick 10-minute pick-me-up, a quick 20-minute energy boost, or a full 30-

minute body detox, chair yoga is available for you, making yoga a comfortable, daily practice. You'll be astonished at how useful and convenient it may be, even from your favorite chair, if you give it a try.

Chapter 7

Chair Yoga Safety Advice

Let's go into the exact safety rules and procedures for chair yoga. We want to make sure you're at ease and acting appropriately.

Things to steer clear of when doing chair yoga.

For instance, leaning too far forward in your chair or slouching might place unnecessary strain on your back. It's important to maintain a straight, intense posture.

Don't push yourself too far, especially in the beginning

When doing chair yoga, it's crucial to do it slowly if you feel any pain. Finally, go slowly while carrying out the procedures. Chair yoga requires you to be aware, so take your time, breathe, and pay attention to your body.

Chair yoga is all about modifying practices to fit your specific requirements. If a position doesn't feel natural, don't force it. Instead, alter it. For instance, if a complete twist is too extreme, a lesser seated twist may be just as effective. Support your body as required using items like cushions or towels. Remember that chair yoga is about your comfort and growth; thus, don't be hesitant to alter poses to suit your unique requirements.

Safety requirements

Always put safety first. Start by choosing a sturdy chair without wheels or armrests and make sure it is on a non-slip surface. Dress comfortably and breathablely, and stay away from loose, possibly tangled accessories. Always see a doctor if you have any concerns about your health before beginning chair yoga. The final and most crucial tip is to pay attention to your body. If something doesn't feel right, stop doing it. The secret to chair yoga is to respect your limitations.

To get the most out of the workout, you may use these chair yoga safety tips and instructions. By avoiding common mistakes, adapting poses to your preferences, and following safety regulations, you can make your chair yoga experience pleasant, safe, and gratifying. So let's be careful and aware; your body will thank you.

Chapter 8

Staying Driven and Reliable

We'll start by discussing how to practice chair yoga regularly and with motivation. Although we all recognize how difficult it may be to keep on schedule, we do have some recommendations.

Know your goals.

With chair yoga, what do you want to accomplish? Maybe there is a little more flexibility, less stress, or just a little more stillness every day. Setting definite, doable objectives may offer you something to strive for and can be a fantastic motivator. It's like having a travel plan for chair yoga.

Chair yoga requires persistence

Just like any other exercise. It's important to create a routine. A quick session every morning or a lengthier session a few times a week can be necessary. To succeed, you must create a habit. It could be a good idea to schedule your chair yoga session the same way you would any other appointment. Also, keep in mind that starting small is acceptable; even a few minutes over time might add up to a big difference.

Joining a Chair Yoga Group or Class

Take into consideration joining a chair yoga group or class if you value responsibility and companionship. You'll have a timetable to stick to, and working in a group may greatly increase motivation. It's a wonderful chance to network with like-minded people and share your chair yoga adventure.

In conclusion

Chair yoga is more than simply exercise; it's like a hidden road to feeling wonderful and full of life, created with our elders in mind. Chair yoga is the way to go whether you're looking for better flexibility, a tranquil moment, or a fun group to join. Why not give it a try and begin

Unlocking Vitality and Aging Gracefully

your path to a better and happier

version of yourself?